GUT INSTINCT

How I healed myself of digestive disease

Kent Petersen

Kent Petersen

Copyright © 2018 by Kent Petersen

The author of this book does not dispense medical advice or prescribe the use of any technique as a form of treatment for physical, emotional, or medical problems without the advice of a physician, either directly or indirectly. The intent of the author is to offer information of a general nature to help you in your quest for well-being. In the event that you use any of the information in this book for yourself, the author assumes no responsibility for your actions.

Table of Contents

Kent Petersen

Mission Statement

To use my knowledge and experience of what helped me remove all evidence of Inflammatory Bowel Disease (IBD) from myself to help as many people as humanly possible.

Dedication & Special Thanks

First, I dedicate this book to anyone with digestive disease and to anyone who is looking to improve their physical condition. May this book bring strength and hope to those who are frustrated and don't know what to do.

Special thanks to my friends, family, and everyone who has supported me and helped me along this journey and a very special thanks to my love, Hezzykat, for her contributions towards naming this book and encouraging me to finally finish it.

Special thanks to Matt Furey, for being a guide and inspiration in my life.

Preface

I have been writing this book over and over again for the last 10+ years. I get to a good stopping point and begin editing the book. During the editing process, I learn new details, new secrets, and new mental shortcuts. Then every time I read over my book I realize I have new information. As I edit, I rewrite the book section by section and never really finish. So, here it is. I finally stopped working on it. It would be wonderful if the book automatically updated itself with the latest knowledge I learn.

A large portion of this book is focused primarily on the mental and mindful aspects of overcoming illness (or anything for that matter), and how changing our mind leads to changes in behaviors, actions, and habits. Many times throughout the book I mention ways to use our mind and imagination to improve digestion. Many of these techniques can be applied to improve numerous conditions. The latter part of the book focuses more on the physical actions we can take to live a healthier life.

This book is not an autobiography and is not intended to share my life story. That portion of the story is included so we all understand where I am coming from.

Success begins with changing yourself

Winning the battle with anything, especially Crohn's Colitis, a severe form of Inflammatory Bowel Disease (IBD), requires a lifestyle change. You will need to improve your thought processes, your mental habits, your physical habits, your activity levels, your understanding of yourself, your diet, your understanding of nutrition, your social interactions, and your environmental experiences. You will need to stay vigilant, be determined, and be positive. Current medical science does not understand the cause of this disease. The disease can be sent into remission with your own power.

Why should you listen to me?

I was diagnosed with IBD and told I would never recover. At my worst, I was having bloody loose bowel movements 50+ times a day with fissures on my anus unable to keep any food in. Now here I am, healthier than I have ever been with one or two solid bowel movements a day and I'm completely pain free. I am baffling doctors with my complete lack of medicine and stunning test results. My last colonoscopy results said, "no evidence of disease"

In addition to that, I have been studying nutrition, fitness, yoga, the mind, medicine, and more for many years. I have worked in a hospital. I have a black belt in Shaolin Kempo. I am a certified yoga teacher. I am

CPR certified. I am excited to share what I have learned with you.

Please consult a doctor before performing any of the following advice. I am not a doctor. I'm not claiming to know medical knowledge.

Why have I written this book?

I originally wrote these tips to help myself. During a particularly rough flare up, I turned to my own written advice. After a relatively short period of time, my flare up reduced. I was thrilled. I realized my advice was sound. I decided I want to help people with IBD and pass on what I learned through trial and error in hopes of saving people some of the pain that I went through.

Since then, I have been sharing my advice with many others and they have been getting positive results too.

Chapter 1:
From Sickness to Lasting Health

Summary of my Story

It all started when I was 20 years old and a Karate instructor, back in the summer of 2003. I was training for my final Brown Belt. In my martial arts style, Shaolin Kempo, this was the belt before Black Belt. I was in incredible shape. Strong, fast, flexible. I was nearly 6'6" and 210 lbs. I never thought something like this could happen to mge.

I was diagnosed with Crohn's disease and ulcerative colitis

I first noticed symptoms months before I thought anything of it. Digestion had been steadily getting worse. Diarrhea had become consistent for at least a couple weeks. I had blood in my stool for at least a couple days.

When I first noticed the diarrhea, I thought nothing of it. Even when it continued for multiple days, I thought nothing of it. Throughout my life I had random bouts of diarrhea and it was never a big deal.

In order to continue working I started using Imodium and various over the counter things to fight the symptoms. This was helpful in masking the symptoms and allowing me to continue my life.

When the bleeding started, I was concerned. Even then, I hoped it would clear up. I made no changes to my life. I figured it would eventually stop but it didn't.

I started making embarrassing messes. Still, I thought nothing of it. I became concerned when I stopped wearing boxers and switched to dark colored briefs. I would wear board shorts and bathing suits because they didn't stain. The situation continued to get worse.

Then, I was literally going to the bathroom every couple hours. I was having at least 5 bowel movements a day. I kept hoping that it would clear up but it did not. The bleeding became severe and I was having trouble sleeping. I really let it get out of hand. I kept trying to keep it to myself.

The night I realized I was sick was truly horrifying. I remember that night so clearly. It was around midnight. I was down at In-N-Out with my friends enjoying one of my favorite burgers when I had to make a mad dash to the bathroom. There was practically no warning. It was extremely urgent. I quickly left my friends and I charged into the restroom, which was relatively clean for a public stall. I turned around, dropped my pants and before I could even sit it exploded out of me. I could feel it with such intensity. I was feeling woozy and light headed. It hurt like a hundred knives stabbing me in the guts. I crumpled over in pain. I cried to myself. After what seemed like forever I opened my eyes and looked about. It had appeared as if someone had been blasted by a shotgun in here. There was blood everywhere. It was on the walls, on the toilet, on the floor. I did the best I could to clean up myself but toilet paper alone would not cut it. I pulled up my pants accepting the loss. I felt bad for the employee who has to clean this mess up. I returned to my friends. Told them I wasn't feeling well and returned home. I didn't let them in on the details. I knew I was in trouble and I would have to get help in the morning.

That night I tossed and turned in unbearable pain. I don't remember sleeping. I must have passed out or blacked out from the pain. I knew I had to go to the doctors in the morning.

My health spiraled out of control as doctors used me like a guinea pig. Test after test drug after drug. They didn't know what was wrong with me and they really wanted to label it.

Medical doctors told me I would never recover

The doctor told me many stories about how stress will affect my health. He told me stories about patients who had relapses on their wedding days. He told stories about patients who worked too hard and caused a flare up. He told me stories about the endless battles. He told me how I will NEVER be completely healthy again. He actually used those words, "You will NEVER be healthy again," I accepted it as true. I didn't understand the significance of these words till much later.

They loaded me up with steroids and other debilitating drugs with minimal results. I was "healthier" to some extent. I tried most of the prescriptions drugs available at the time, including, Prednisone (a corticosteroid),

6-MP (6-mercaptopurine is typically a cancer medication that interferes with the growth and spread of cells in the body. It is used in fighting IBD that has not responded to other drugs), and Asacol (aka Mesalamine, an aspirin-like anti-inflammatory drug), Remicade and Humira (both are TNF alpha inhibitor. Remicade contains rat). Frustratingly, all of these yielded minimal (if any) results.

Doctors destroyed my hope

My doctor insisted I will have symptoms for life. At that moment, I accepted this as true. I believed the professionals. I figured the doctors know best. Even though, the doctor said I would NEVER be healed and that it can come back at ANY time. The doctor did not paint an optimistic picture for me.

The doctor insisted that diet plays NO role in fixing

IBD symptoms and suggested we played with the dosages of the drugs. He said most people responded to drugs and the drugs should be able to induce a remission. I wanted to live a normal life. I trusted him. No doctor ever found the correct dosage or medication that would induce a lasting remission.

Even the dietician who specializes in IBD did not have an answer

I did what I feel most people would do in my situation, I gave up hope. I didn't even attempt to fix it. Why would I? The doctors and experts said diet didn't matter. They didn't tell me about any behavioral changes that I could make which may help. Instead, they said medicine was the only solution and the drugs were not helping anymore.

The lows were very low

At my worse, I was in terrible shape. I had lost over 50 pounds, I was nearly 6'6" and I weighed less than 150 lbs. My bowel movement count was through the roof. I was going to the bathroom every 15 minutes. Every stool had blood, mucus, and chunks of intestines. I was weaker than ever. I had constant intense cramps. During this time, I was literally crippled, walking was excruciating due to my skin splitting open around the anus due to frequent wiping and passing of stools. Doctors called it anal fissures. This continued on for months.

Current medical science didn't know how to manage this disease for me. Every doctor I went to said the condition was permanent and I would be on drugs for life. I didn't like that answer.

Tired of doctors and drugs not working, I decided to change my approach. I decided to manage it myself. I was sick and tired of being sick and tired. The transformation fully began.

The path was challenging, especially at first

As the months and years went by, I learned what worked and what did not work for me. I wrote down my advice and my processes to help remember what worked for me. With this information, I could minimize the worst moments and maximize the best moments. I wrote down everything, including what worked out well and what made me feel awful. I repeated the beneficial stuff and avoided the things that hindered me. This information became the foundation for this book.

I began to change

I learned which foods I could tolerate and digest better. I learned that some foods were digested best at different times of the day. I learned that certain foods were harder to digest when mixed with other foods. I learned the complexities and intricacies of eating and the composition of what we are eating. I learned about chemicals and pH levels in our bodies. I learned how stress, including but not limited to mental, physical, and emotional puts a strain on the body and reduces digestion and slows healing. I studied exercises I could perform when I was weak and helped with digestion. Such as inversions, breathing exercises, yoga, and walking.

I started with simple breathing exercises and mild slow movements. This in turn would lift my spirits and cleanse my mind. I performed them regularly.

With exercise came peace of mind and soon happiness. My health steadily improved from there.

I took life very easy. One day at a time. I felt like I started a new life. My thinking, my habits, and my way of being changed. I emphasized relaxing and being calm. I encouraged healthy eating and created a mellow environment. I was able to see the stress I was under. I learned to release it.

This new me is a great wonderful enjoyable version of me. I sleep better. I hold on to less stress and drop stress easier and quicker. I enjoy exercise and I keep getting stronger. My habits and my thoughts changed. With persistence and consistency my new preferred habits and ways of thinking became a part of me.

There were ups and downs but overall I became

healthier, clearer, and made preferred choices easier. My symptoms slowly faded away.

I became healthier than ever. I could go out with no concern of an unexpected bowel movement for the first time in years. I stopped looking for bathrooms every time I entered somewhere new. I continued to steadily improve.

As my health returned, so did the burning desire to be strong again. The intensity of my exercise routines increased. The food I ate was as nutrient dense as possible.

When my health slipped and flare ups intensified, I would return to the advice and notes I wrote myself with great success.

There came a moment when my guts completely

stopped hurting.

After a nearly a decade, I finally stopped hurting!

Yes, I'm repeating myself. This is amazing to me.

I noticed that my insides don't feel bad anymore. My guts do not hurt. They don't ache. There are no cramps. The left side feels just as good as the right now. For the first time in 8 years I FEEL GREAT. I am pain free again!

To see if I was great according to western medical science, I went back to a gastroenterologist for the first time in years. I showed him 40+ pages of my old medical information and talked about how wonderful I was feeling. He was surprised I did this without meds and called the healing a spontaneous remission. I chuckled and said "It wasn't spontaneous. I have been working hard at making lifestyle changes and maintaining my health." I listed off a few of the things that I have been doing, like cutting fast food and soda from my diet, daily exercise, meditation, using cannabis, and keeping a positive state of mind. He then told me to keep doing what I'm doing. He encouraged me to keep smoking weed and he was very happy for me. Apparently I was supposed to get a colonoscopy every 2-3 years. I was well overdue. The doctor wanted to take a look inside to see how well I was really doing.

Surprisingly, it was a good experience. The lab results I got were exactly what I hoped they would be. First, I compared the old archived pictures that I have to the new pictures. My intestines looked phenomenal. The lack of inflammation and bright red sections are profoundly obvious. Then I read the notes. "No evidence of active Crohn's disease or ulcer in the entire colon and terminal ileum"

To summarize: No signs of disease in my intestines. Go me!

I overcame the odds. Doctors told me my insides would be scarred for life. Now there is no evidence of scarring. Doctors told me I would be drugged for life. Now, I don't take any meds. I took it into my own hands and listened to my internal doctor. I followed my own advice that I knew deep inside, is best for me.

Currently, I'm in the best shape of my life. This experience has been so transformational for me I feel very inspired to share my knowledge and wisdom to help give ideas to anyone who also wants to overcome bleak odds. I am excited to share some of what I have learned.

Chapter 2:

You Will Achieve Anything you Focus your Mind on

What you think of yourself is what your self will become

Consider this point of view to unlock the potential power of your mind. The idea is that your mind and your thoughts create who you are and what you do. It is easy to realize this if you notice your thoughts become your words. Your words become your actions. Your actions become your habits. Your habits create your character. You character creates who you are.

With this idea in mind it's easy to see how healthy positive thoughts will create a healthy positive person. It is also easy to see how healthy positive thoughts and being a healthy positive person are essential to creating a healthy positive body.

Decide that you *CAN* be healthy again

Once you understand the previous perspective. The first and most important thing you MUST do is decide that it is in fact possible to be healthy again. If you do not think you CAN be healthy, you will prove yourself right. If you think there is a chance that you can be healthy again the doors of possibility can open. Have faith in your body and its healing capacity. Your body wants to exist in a healthy state.

Your cells are constantly regenerating. All you need to do is supply proper nutrition, habits, thoughts, and actions to allow the body to heal.

You MUST believe it is possible before you can allow the healing to take place. If you are having a hard time believing this idea, take a moment and imagine what it would be like to have better digestion. Imagine the goal with as many vivid details as you can. Make the image in your mind's eye so detailed and positive that you automatically smile. Once you have that clear vivid image or feeling of this possibility and what it would be like, tell yourself, "I *can* be healthy again." If saying this makes you upset in any way you do not believe yet.

It helped me to imagine how great the possibility of being healthy feels. Keep repeating this mental exercise every day or as often as possible until you believe that you *can* be healthy again. You need to accept that you CAN be healthy before healing can take place.

For a few years, I thought I would never be healthy again. All the doctors I spoke with told me this was a lifelong illness. They said I would have to deal with the disease forever and I just need to learn to accept it and learn to cope with it. They assured me there were no permanent fixes. This became a limiting belief for me. As long as I believed this, there was no way I could be healthy again. I would not take the appropriate actions to move in a healthy direction because I believed the actions would not help. Changing the mind to accept the possibility of health is the first and most important step to greater health

Decide that you *WILL* be healthy again no matter what

After realizing that health is possible, the next most important step to take is making the firm decision that you will be healthy again. Do not accept failure. Know deep inside that you will succeed.

For me, knowing that I will do something has a lot more powerful energy and feeling behind it than knowing I can do something.

Have your mind set on the goal of being healthy with a burning desire. This will align your actions, habits, and thoughts. All three must be congruent and aligned before serious change can begin. If you are not congruent it's because you don't really believe it yet. Make sure you KNOW that you can be healthier than you are now.

As soon as you KNOW that you WILL be healthy again you will automatically begin to make the proper adjustments in your life to achieve this. You will begin to see more clearly the choices that will help you progress towards your goal of lasting health.

First, I had to realize that I could be healthy again despite what the professionals were telling me. Then, I had to make up my mind and decide that no matter what I *will* be healthy again. I had to take a step back from the doctors, the dietitians, and the experts who had no positive advice for me. I had to look outside the box and adjust my mind and my perspective to accept that these experts are just people they do not know everything. They cannot feel how I feel.

Once I made up my mind that I will be healthy

again the appropriate changes began. I was determined to not let disease hinder my life. You could do the same.

Often having a strong determination to achieve something will take you much farther than you originally thought possible.

Think healthy thoughts

Behavior and thought patterns can create psychosomatic diseases. We can use the same concept in reverse by focusing on health and vitality to cure diseases. This is like a placebo effect that you create yourself. Limit unhealthy thoughts and replace them with thoughts of health and strength.

Healthy people don't think about how sick they are. Sick people do. If you want to be a healthy person you need to start thinking like a healthy person. Instead of spending all of your time thinking about how sick you are, focus on positive things like what currently excites you or what you can do to become healthier.

When I relapsed, I would often bring up how sick I was in conversation and I would talk about all the things I used to be able to do and could not anymore. I talked about how much of a challenge conquering the disease was. My mind was filled with negativity and excuses for failure. My relapse did not end until I changed these thoughts. I needed to stop reminding myself how much pain I was in. I needed to remind myself that progress takes action. Take it one step at a time. Keep the positive thoughts of success and let go of the thoughts of negativity.

Use the power of imagination to succeed

Sometimes it's hard to believe you can get to the end goal of lasting health. You can use the power of your mind's imagination to help you.

It has been shown in numerous studies that the mind cannot tell the difference between something that is real and something that has been vividly imagined with as much detail as possible. Let that thought sink in for a moment. The power of this statement is vast. It implies that if you imagine something with as much realistic detail as possible, according to your mind, it is just as good as actually doing it.

Use this idea and use your imagination as a powerful tool for projecting and testing future possibilities. You can imagine any aspect of any detail. If you can allow yourself to imagine what it would be like to be healthy then you can begin to feel the change take place inside.

Take a moment to imagine what better health would feel like. In your mind's eye, create the healthy feelings you want to have. Make the details as vivid as you can. Consider how you would feel? How much water you would drink? What kind of foods you would eat? How much pain are you not in? How tall would you stand? The more real you can make the image the easier it will be to attain.

At first this task of imagining what you want may seem difficult or silly. As with everything, the more you practice the better you will become. In time, you may find using your imagination to be not only simple but enjoyable.

As a practice exercise, I like to spend a few minutes every day imagining what it would be like to be healthy. In a positive mindset, I vividly imagine all the enjoyable things I would be doing if I was not hindered by illness. I imagine and FEEL the positive feelings that I will have. Once I am filled with a positivity I go about my day knowing that the actions I take will eventually lead me to my goal.

As you become more connected with using your imagination, you may want to try another mental exercise. Take a few minutes to focus on how much progress you have made. Imagine the feeling of progression. If progress is minimal or if you want to really boost your progression, you can imagine the progress that you WILL make. Make it as real and vivid as possible. Encompass as many senses as you can.

Use your imagination to feel the end result you prefer.

Example Imagination Exercise:

In your imagination see yourself the way you prefer to be. Imagine yourself with perfect health. See the cells of your body regenerating. Feel the cells regenerating. Hear the self-talk you are giving yourself as your body restores itself. As this imaginary experience is practiced you are actively healing your body, the more vivid the scene, the more powerful and real the effect. The more we practice this imaginary experience the easier it becomes. Try it out and see for yourself.

Check your self-image then boost it with your imagination

Your self-image is your personal idea of yourself.

Everyone has a self-image. If you think of yourself, you are checking your self-image.

Take a moment to check in with the self-image and imagine the kind of person you think you are. Is this an image of someone who is dependent on other people or is it an image of someone who can solve their own problems? Is this the image of someone who is always sickly or someone who is becoming healthier? Is this the image of someone who makes excuses or gets things done? Is this the kind of person who belittles themselves for mistakes or gets right back in there and tries again?

Be the kind of person that looks out for themselves and makes healthy choices. Be the kind of person who doesn't care about peer pressure and do what is right for you. Be the kind of person who makes positive changes and establishes positive habits.

Then the rest will be easy.

Use the power of your Imagination. See yourself being the kind of person you want to be. Imagine it in as much vivid detail as possible. Then take action.

Easier done than said

Anytime things seem indescribable, overwhelming, out of control, or impossible remember the mantra "Easier done than said." Often words are inept in describing feelings and experiences. Realize anything is as complicated as you make it out to be. If you think the process is simple it will be. On the other hand, If you think the process is complicated it will be. Often times, the act of doing is far easier than explaining as long as you know what you want. You do not have to understand why things work. Just know that they will as long as you continue to give directed positive effort. Give your best effort in the direction of health and know your health will improve. With this idea in mind, simplify as often as possible and reduce unneeded complications from your life.

Chapter 3:
Your Mood, Attitude, and Mental State, Affects your Health

Unhappiness breeds pain and irritation

When I was sickly it was very easy to become extremely unhappy and irritable. There are many things to be unhappy about. I found the more unhappy I became, the worse my health became. The more my health tanked, the more irritable I became. The more unhappy I became, the more aware of the pain I became. The more in tune with the negativity I became, the more negative I became, the less I would care about my goals of health.

When feeling this way, I found I would fall back on old habits of consuming junk food, like candy bars and ice cream. As my misery grew, I found I did not care about my health and I cared less about my goals. The downward spiral would continue. The unhappiness would breed more pain and irritation. The pain and irritation would breed more unhappiness and turn into more poor choices and poor habits. Unhappiness is a slippery spiral slope and when you start sliding down it, it is easy to get caught up in the misery.

Be aware of the cycle and break it. Focus on the positive aspects, like knowing it is possible to heal.

Be excited to change and break free of misery.

Be positive, happy, and excited about being healthy and well

A happy, excited, positive attitude has many benefits. You may have noticed that when you are in this state of being, you focus on more positivity. Your outlook becomes more positive and you are drawn to more positivity. People who are more positive will prefer to spend more time with you. It becomes easier to make a greater effort to take care of yourself and make more positive decisions. You will have more fun in your undertakings.

When you are happy, excited, and positive, your body will naturally release more endorphins which will help you feel better, hurt less, heal faster, and feel good. When you work with excitement, tedious activities may seem fun again. Hard work may become easier to perform and you will be more willing to perform it. When you are excited about a goal and have a positive attitude, you are more likely to take positive action. It will be easier to be consistent and eager to push on. Consistent positive action will quickly bring you to your goal. If you are excited about the steps you need to take it will be easier to take the necessary steps more often.

Make being healthy your exciting goal of the day and be excited about the changes that will take place. Be excited knowing that you will improve as long as you keep taking positive action. Be fired up about health. Let the thoughts bring a smile to your face. Feel the excitement deep inside. The more excited you are the easier and quicker the results will come.

As you become more positive, negativity will melt away from you. You may notice negative events and activities affect you less and you may be able to see them as simpler, easier, or less bothersome.

Reduce stress levels and relax your way to health

Emotions have powerful effects on your health. When you are feeling stress, fear, anxiety, and worry, the sympathetic nervous system activates and inhibits digestion. This leaves food sitting around in your digestive tract for longer periods of time with minimal nutrient absorption which promotes an improper bacteria balance. For optimal health and digestion avoid these feelings, especially before eating and sleeping. Avoid confrontation especially during a flare up. Avoid stressful activities. Life is too short to live stressed out.

If stress is unavoidable (and it often is) take a moment to relax and take a few deep breaths while working on the stressful task. Take the time to let go of negative feelings and anything that no longer serves you. Use your imagination to grab all the stress, negativity, and confrontation that is currently bothering you, take it down to the trash can and throw it in. Then imagine the garbage truck picking it up and taking it away. Feel it leaving your being. Feel it leaving your body. Feel it leaving your soul.

Relaxing goes a long way in helping your body digest food. Your digestive system functions best when you are in a calm and relaxed state. When you are relaxed, the parasympathetic nervous system activates. The parasympathetic nervous system is responsible for resting activities including nourishing, healing, and regeneration of the body and digestion activities including salivation, urination, digestion, and defecation. With this in mind it is easy to see that your body heals faster when you are relaxed. Relaxation is key to reducing stress and promoting healing.

When I was calm, relaxed, or happy my guts felt calm and relaxed. My symptoms would reduce and they were easier to manage. When I was depressed, upset, angry or bitter, the day seemed much worse. Everything hurt more and bowel movements per day increased dramatically.

Find activities that make you feel more relaxed and perform them daily. Take the time to make sure you are in a calm relaxed state. I recommend yoga, walking, and tuning into your breathing to reduce stress levels.

Maintain a balanced objective mind

To allow yourself to use your best judgment and make the best possible choices based on this particular moment you must maintain a balanced mind. You must accept the reality of the situation as it is, not as you wish it to be. Be aware of your mental state.

If you notice that you are feeling negative feelings or thinking negative thoughts, avoid getting caught up in the pity party or following the typical cycle of making poor choices. Instead, recognize these thoughts, feelings, and sensations. See the moment objectively as it really is then take the best action to improve the situation. Do not let the bad times warp your perception or throw you off track.

For example, I ate my favorite food that does not

agree with me and I end up in the bathroom in serious pain. In the past, I would typically crumple over and cry and wonder why this is happening to me and not everyone else. These thoughts do not lead to solutions, only an upset mind. When you recognize the reality of the situation, the favorite food caused this suffering, then it is easier to change your course of action to be something beneficial. Perhaps start some deep breathing exercises to help digestion. Then next time you are selecting your food, you may select something different to eat knowing which food caused this discomfort.

Remember, it's not your fault

Do not dwell on the potential mistakes that might have brought you to the situation you are in now. Medical science has not figured out the cause of many diseases, including inflammatory bowel diseases. Dwelling can exacerbate symptoms and does little to induce healing.

Even though, it is not your fault, you can start taking positive action to help speed up the recovery.

Never give up

The road to recovery can be difficult. It's a slippery slope with many ups and downs. Trying to heal yourself on your own can be discouraging at times. There can be many situations that could make most people want to give up.

Sometimes it seems like no progress is made. My improvement is rarely constant when gauged on a day to day basis. I didn't let it hinder me. I noticed, over the course of many months, the results were clearly improving.

Whatever happens, keep improving yourself. As long as you consistently and continuously do your best to improve your health with a positive attitude, you will continue to improve. The healing process is toughest in the beginning, when you are breaking old negative habits and releasing old limiting beliefs.

Once new healthy positive habits form and expansive beliefs are accepted, the battle becomes much easier as your new habits and beliefs automatically propel you to greater health. Have patience. It may take time to change. Have faith in yourself. You can do anything you set your mind to.

It took me 7 years to induce my first lasting remission. I learned many things about myself along the way. If I gave up before this, I may have never learned how to maintain my health like I now can or write this book. With the knowledge I learned on this journey, I was able to induce my second lasting remission in only 7 months. This refined my knowledge even more.

There were many times when I found the foods I ate gave me inconsistent results. I was making embarrassing messes and spending all day in the bathroom. It can be tough at times. I know I went through it. It can definitely wear you down, if you allow it.

Every time I feel like quitting my better feeling lifestyle choices and reverting to my previous lifestyle, I remind myself why I wanted the healthy positive change in the first place. I remind myself of the life I have or had before and imagine the life I am working on now. Decide what is more important to you and act upon your decision with all your effort.

When my symptoms were at their most severe I had lost over 50 pounds from my normal weight. I weighed 145 lbs. I was going to the bathroom every 15 minutes, I couldn't walk because the extreme frequency lead to fissures around my anus, and I was weaker than ever.

Even then, I didn't give up. I did not consider my current situation permanent. I knew deep inside, my health would eventually improve if I continued with doing things that made me feel better. I thought that it may be possible to recover from this disease. It turned out I was right.

Good health is the greatest gift of life

When you are healthy with no ailments, pain free with no aches, have an active and powerful mind, and have a strong and flexible body, it is easy to enjoy the gift of life. With good health, life is more enjoyable. With good health, it is easier to express positivity to those who are around you. When you have the gift of health, savor the moment. Take some time to feel how wonderful this moment feels and note the changes in your perception. Take advantage of your health and do something you enjoy. Enjoy every moment. You never know what kind of challenges life will throw your way.

Remember the negativity that comes with poor health including aches and pains, scattered thoughts and doubt, stiffness and injuries, weakness and disease. With poor health you are more irritable. With poor health, you are straining the ones you love.

After the symptoms began to dissipate and I restored my health for the first time, I started slacking and going back to my old ways of thinking and acting. I took my hard work for granted. I thought I was done. I did not realize that living healthy is a lifestyle change and "everyone else" is on their way to sickness and disease. I did not realize yet, that my old behavior and habits patterns is what created the situation I was in. At this time, I thought I didn't need to have a healthy lifestyle anymore.

As I took my health and my hard work for granted, the symptoms started to return. The symptoms escalated and snowballed out of control very quickly. Suddenly, I had a full relapse.

The transition from good health to poor health is very humbling. The transition back from poor health to good health is very empowering. Appreciate your health. Do whatever it takes to create lasting health. It is an investment well worth the time. Take action on healthy choices. Experience the results you create. Use the results as fuel to inspire yourself to keep going.

Remember the past to motivate you now

Whenever I need motivation to overcome unhealthy desires, I take a moment to remember how terrible this situation can get. I remember the horrible burning pain. I remember the sleepless nights spent crying in agony. I remember the constant barrage of diarrhea. I remember all the times I messed myself. I remember all the blood. I remember all the times I was knee deep in it trying to clean up. I remember all the times that I let someone down because I was tied up in the bathroom. I take all those horrible feelings and I ask myself. Is it worth it?

I compare how painful and horrible I felt to how great I could feel now. I could be free of constant pain. I could be free of urgently rushing to the bathroom. I could eat nutritious foods that I want without fear of repercussion. I could sleep through the night again. I could be more free of limitations regarding what I can do or accomplish.

Remembering that I have risen above these issues improved my state of being. Remembering how I was before the disease is my motivation for moving forward and avoiding regression. I do not want to fall back into a sickly state of being. No one deserves a life of pain or suffering.

Listen to your inner doctor

When I listen to how I feel, my life synchronizes with my feelings. With a positive attitude, I receive a positive life. I do whatever is conducive to my health and my happiness. I follow my excitement. I listen to my inner doctor. As I do this, I become much healthier with wonderful results.

Learn to calibrate yourself. Ask yourself simple empowering questions and wait for the answer. Questions like, "Am I excited to act on this right now?" or "How does this generate more health and happiness in my life?"

Check in with yourself and make sure that what you are doing feels right for you. After every decision or action be aware of how you feel. If you are not sure, take the moment to tune in to yourself and see where you may lead yourself next. Maybe write down some notes about how you feel and what you have been doing.

Try it for yourself, listen to your inner doctor that already knows what to do. Trust yourself, you know yourself better than anyone else knows you.

Thinking and knowing

Thoughts are limited by the amount of time they take to process. For example if you are talking to yourself in your thoughts you are limited to the time it takes to get the words out and you are limited by your vocabulary. Thinking in images is a bit faster. Images can convey a more in depth thought than mere words in less time. It is also possible to visualize things you can't describe. You can create rich, vivid and powerful thoughts by encompassing many senses.

Your mind can perceive quicker than even that. Beyond thinking is knowing. There are many occurrences when you know something to be true. You do not need to think about the circumstance.

For example if you come up to a ledge of a cliff you know that if you slip off you will get hurt. No time is needed to think over the situation. The knowledge is there and you innately know what it means.

You know when you are in pain. You know when you are healthy. You know when you are happy. You know when you are not. Spend less time thinking and more time paying attention to what you confidently know.

For example, I knew when I was not in complete remission. I still felt the pain burn deep down inside. The lower left quadrant of my intestines still ached. Sometimes, I would think to myself that this was good enough but I knew I could feel better.

Avoid over thinking, it may fill you with doubt and consumes needless energy.

Go beyond thought, perceive and know.

Chapter 4:
Create New Habits to Automate your Preferable Lifestyle

Transform to a healthier lifestyle

Doing whatever it is you are doing now is giving you the results in your life that you are getting now. If you want different results in your life do something different.

If you want your guts to be healthier make

healthier decisions when it comes to eating, drinking, stress management, sleep habits, or anything else. Permanently fixing health issues is not just a simple one time action. It's something you are going to keep fine tuning, making it a part of your daily life. Make being healthy a part of your self-image. Become the kind of person who makes healthy choices.

At first, this may seem overwhelming. You may have a lot of negative habits that you will need to overcome. The good news is that once you start making a lifestyle change and break the old bad habits, the new healthy habits that you replaced them with will begin to automatically propel you to a healthy victory. Once you start getting the momentum rolling it becomes easier and easier to keep getting better and better healthier results. Avoid searching for the magic bullet that will solve all your problems. Put in the effort to change who you are. It will be worth it.

Any action taken may form into a habit

Any action repeated is more likely to form into a habit. I define habits as unconsciously triggered personal patterns. The habits you have determine actions you take when you are unaware or falling back into a pattern. This is very valuable information that can be used to your advantage.

Yogis say it takes approximately 40 consecutive days of consecutive action to break an old habit. Continued work on the habit will reinforce it and make it stronger and more natural. If continued for about 90 days you have formed a new habit. Some of the more deep rooted negative habits that have been ingrained over the years may require more diligence to replace.

Create positive habits to automate good behavior

In my opinion, anytime spent creating positive habits is time well spent. When good behavior becomes a habit, the behavior will activate automatically when triggered. Creating good habits will free up time, energy, and mental space that can be used to work on creating more positive habits. Create the habit of creating positive preferable habits.

Take the time to eliminate negative wasteful habits including eating right before bed, calling yourself names, eating unhealthy foods, drinking soda, self-doubt, expressing negativity, insulting others, putting yourself down, by asking the question, "Why did I do that?"

To remove negative habits, you must bring the unconscious action or habit trigger into your awareness. As you observe this moment, take a different action than you normally would. Replace the unwanted action with the action you want to do. Each time you repeat this will reinforce the new habit.

Make all positive routines habits. Become the kind of person who has a habit of making good habits. Become the kind of person who has the habit of breaking bad habits. Mastering these two habits will take you far.

Be mindful of your habits

It's important to keep your mind in check. What you think guides you to the actions you take. The actions you take will form into the habits you have. A positive mind will generate positive habits. A negative mind will generate negative habits. Time spent forming and imagining positive habits will help generate and reinforce them. The same is true for the negative.

As vividly as you can, imagine yourself forming the habit you wish to have. Focus on how performing this new habit feels. Allow the positive feelings to consume you. Then do it.

Take it one day at a time

Think to yourself, "I am going to be healthier today than I was yesterday." Then take the proper action to make it true. Make it a goal. Everyday take at least one action to improve your wellbeing. If you keep at it you will have this as a habit and healing is inevitable.

Develop discipline easily when excited

If you are genuinely excited about whatever you are doing you will have all the self-discipline you need to continue. When excited, you will be ready and willing to work hard and be happy to perform well. When excited, you will be eager for more. When excited, time becomes irrelevant and you will be able to put in long hours with ease and focus. The more excited you are the easier the task is to perform. Act on your highest excitement for an exciting fulfilling life.

Have excitement for a lifestyle change. As I became more and more excited about healthy living, improvement came automatically. Self-discipline developed itself. Making positive choices became easier. My health steadily improved. I became healthier and healthier, stronger and stronger.

Accomplish goals faster when excited

Accomplishing a challenging or seemingly impossible goal takes daily conscious effort. To ensure success pick meaningful goals that you actually want to accomplish. Pick meaningful goals that draw you to them. Pick a goal that gets you excited now. Do something toward this goal EVERY day.

My goal is creating lasting health. I make a conscious effort to do one thing toward restoring my health EVERY day. Some days I want to eat better, other days, I sleep more. Often, I would spend a few minutes and imagine what it feels like to be feel better and be healthy.

Chapter 5:
Give your Body what it Needs

Know your body's needs

The human body recovers best when it is in a relaxed state, receives a healthy balance of nutritious foods, gets plenty of mineral water, breathes fresh oxygen, participates in some physical movement, and receives a good night sleep.

Physically move your body around

Provide your body with exercise to keep your organs, muscles, and tissues active and functioning at an optimal level and allow blood flow to each area. Use all of your body parts. Stretch out to allow your body to fully extend. Take time to relax after. Breathe deeply to improve oxygen flow.

Maintain a well-balanced diet that feels right

When I was trying out different diets, I had become horribly malnourished from the intense training for my black belt and the lack of well-balanced nutritious foods. I was dehydrated from sweating during training and frequency of bowel movements. I did not consume enough water, salt, and electrolytes to make up the loss. My body just could not keep up with my actions. I felt weak but I pushed on expecting the advice of others to help me.

If you are following a diet or following advice and you feel weak and feel like your body feels worse, slow down what you are doing and evaluate yourself. Figure out why they recommend the diet or advice and figure out why it's not working out for you. Learn for yourself. Be a scientist.

To make a diet well-balanced, avoid foods with no nutritional value and foods that are packed full of chemicals, additives, or preservatives. If it is not achieved through eating a nutritional food, take herbal supplements to maintain a proper balance of nutrition.

Now I know, I could have maintained a well-balanced diet and drank more mineral water. I could have paid attention to my body when I was exercising and training. I could have avoided over doing it. I thought the old adage "No pain. No gain." was true. I disagree. Now I believe, "Slow and steady wins the race."

Get plenty of rest and sleep
Sleep is good for you, your mind, and your body

This one may be difficult right now but you want to get as much uninterrupted sleep as possible. Your body does most of its healing and cell repairing when your body is relaxing during a good night sleep. It has been shown that the body delays wound healing with sleep deprivation.

Sleep rests your body and your mind. Sleep allows you to slip into a relaxed mental state. This will allow you to think clearer, maintain a positive happy attitude, become excited more easily, allows your mind to be able to process the previous day, and prepares our mind for the next day. Physically, sleep will allow your body the chance to reduce tension and restores damaged cells.

Most adults need between 6 - 8 hours of sleep a night. You will most likely need more if you are currently healing. I had noticeable health improvements once I could start sleeping 4+ hours at once. My healing really started taking off once I could sleep through the night. Sleep as much as you need to. When I was very sickly (50+ bowel movements a day), I would require 12+ hours of sleep to feel refreshed. In addition to that I would take multiple naps throughout the day.

Make sure you get enough sleep. The healthier I become the less I feel I need to sleep. The more I reduce stress from my life, the less I feel I need to sleep.

Create good habits that will help allow you sleep through the night. Controlling your sleep habits may help induce longer periods of sleep. Try sleeping at the same time every day to get in the habit of sleeping. Try to get some physical activity in during the day to increase sleep efficacy. Avoid food that may energize you and prevent sleep before bed. Do whatever it takes to get a good night sleep.

Give your body time to heal

Healing wounds takes time. Internal wounds, like your digestive system, are no different. It takes time for your body to heal from the damage it has suffered. This may not be something that will go away in a single night. It may take some time, patience, focus, and self-discipline. My first remission took 7 years to induce and lasted for a few months. My 2nd remission took 7 months and lasted for about 2 years. I was applying everything I learned the first time around. My 3rd remission took 6 months to be up and running and only a few months from then to be in the best shape of my life. Be prepared for a long fight but do everything you can to make it quick.

Yoga to strengthen and restore our body

I found yoga to be very helpful for building up core strength and healing our organs. Yoga builds muscle and strength around the tender areas and supports them. Yoga teaches us how to move our body in alignment with strength and ease. Yoga teaches us to relax injured areas so they can heal. Yoga teaches us how to break up fascia and scar tissue and rejuvenate the body. Yoga develops our self-awareness. It brings an increase in blood flow to the injured area and assists in circulation, and helps promote healing. Yoga is great for healing. It helps you learn, know, and understand your limits. Keep it slow and simple. Pushing yourself too hard could cause increased pain, slow healing, and increased bowel movements.

If exercise increases pain or urgency you are exercising too hard or too much

When I was first hit with this disease I was a martial arts instructor. I found the intense exercises that we did and the physical impact we experienced were often too much for my guts. Being hard on my body would force me to spend a lot of time with loose stools in the bathroom.

When my guts were soft and tender they would hurt from light physical touch. I learned that light low impact exercise such as walking, stretching, yoga, and deep breathing, were best during and after a flare up.

As I recovered, my aches and pains began to dull and fade. I could tolerate more. I would slowly increase the intensity of my exercising based on what I could do that day. As the pain reduced the urgency reduced I was able to introduce more exercises. If at any point the pain or urgency increased from exercise, I would reduce the intensity or cut back on or stop doing the exercise that caused it.

Keep your body slightly warm

In my experience, I tend to have more digestion

issues when my body is cold. As my body becomes more cold and stiff, my organs cramp, become stiff, and spasm. As my body warms up it reduces pain and cramps. I like to keep my body's temperature at a comfortable or slightly warm temperature. This gives me the best comfort and digestive results.

During a flare up, being hot is hard on my body and may exacerbate my symptoms. For me, digestive problems and frequency would increase when I was too hot such as after intense exercise, during a fever, or spending time in the sauna.

For me a chilly breeze would increase bathroom trip frequency. Rainy days would cause extra pain and discomfort if I were to stay wet and cold. A warm day would leave me feeling good.

In my experience, there are simple methods for

adjusting your body temperature including taking a shower, eating food, drinking tea, or specific breathing techniques.

Taking a shower is a good way to modify my body temperature. A warm shower will warm my body up quick. I like to take an extra moment when showering to run warm water over my abdominal region to soften the cramping and relax the area.

When I eat colder food my body becomes colder. Eating warmer food warms up my body. I found I digest things best when they are near my body temperature. For me, cold foods are harder to digest than warm foods. Cold water, ice cubes, ice cream, and other cold foods, would put a huge strain on my digestive system. I would avoid putting ice cubes in my drinking water when I was having digestion problems.

Physically exercise your body in some way daily

This means EVERY day. You don't have to do a lot. Just do something physical. Spend at least 1 minute a day doing something that moves your body around. Don't give the excuse that there is no time for that. Everyone can make time for at least 1 minute. As you build the habit to exercise you may find that you enjoy this and you may want to increase the amount of time you work out. Work your way up to an amount of exercise that you find comfortable each day.

Try exercising at different times of the day until you find what feels right for you. I found that exercising in the morning right after my first bowel movement made the rest of my day feel better.

If exercising is challenging due to injury modify the exercises in a way that makes them easy enough to perform in your current state.

If exercising is impossible due to injury, spend the minute imagining yourself exercising in the most exciting way possible as vividly as possible. Allow the sensation to fill you up inside and truly FEEL as if you are happily exercising right now and notice the effect this has on you.

Try different exercises to find out what you enjoy. Light exercise like yoga, walking, or swimming is recommended, especially if you are just starting out. If that is too much you could practice deep breathing, sitting up straight, or standing with proper alignment.

Deep breathing alone has made many weak people strong and many sick people well

Deep breathing gets more oxygen in your system which helps your body heal. It increases blood flow which brings nutrient rich blood into various areas of the body and moves toxins out. Deep breathing will help you think clearer. It gives energy, vitality, and strength. It will tune up your body and tune you into your body's needs. It will help you listen to how you feel. I cannot emphasize enough how helpful deep breathing is for me.

To breathe deeply, breathe from your diaphragm. Inhale deeply and imagine the air going all the way down to your toes. Push out your belly and expand it fully, allow this space to fill with air. Allow your lungs to expand laterally like wings. Allow the air to rise up and fill your chest and throat. Imagine energy filling your body. Exhale fully and imagine the old toxic air leaving your system. During the exhale, pull your belly button in towards your spine. Breathe like this as often as possible. Make belly breathing a habit.

Deep breathing with gentle abdominal squeezing

This technique has consistently helped with balancing my digestion. It helps balance an irritated bowel. Gently perform this technique in a calm relaxed state and only continue if it feels good. If internal bleeding is present or if this causes pain, do not do this exercise until after the pain and bleeding has subsided.

Inhale deeply and fully. Feel your chest expand as described above. When you are full of air gently squeeze your abdomen and slowly exhale. Squeeze and exhale until you are completely out of air. Inhale and catch your breath. Repeat. Performing this 3 - 10 times always does the trick for me. I like to do this every time I'm stuck in the bathroom to help move my stools along.

Improve your posture

Good posture is good for digestion. It opens up the pathways and allows your body to perform peristalsis more efficiently. Sit and stand up tall as often as possible, especially when eating. If you are not sure what good posture feels like practice by placing your shoulders, hips, and skull flat against a wall. Push your feet into the earth when you stand. Make sure there is even weight in both feet. Lift your rib cage up. Allow your shoulder blades to flatten on your back. Chin even with the floor. The spine is in alignment from sacrum to base of the skull. Crown of the head lifts up towards the sky.

Push your feet into the ground when you walk. Press evenly through the inner and outer side of the foot as the weight shifts with your stride.

When you sit have even weight in both sit bones and press them down into the seat to create lift in your body.

Yoga will help reshape your posture and build your internal awareness. Daily practice is beneficial. Once good posture becomes a habit you won't have to think about it anymore and there are tremendous benefits.

Chapter 6:
Mindful Consumption Concepts

Every body is different

This was a challenging section for me to write. Originally, I had a section full of various recipes but I decided it's an ever changing answer and this is unique for each individual. My diet varies from moment to moment. Many factors affect what foods your body may need and desire. Consider a few factors that may affect your dietary choices. Are you hot or cold? Are you aware of your sensitivities? Do you have the flu? Do you have allergies? How much do you weigh? How active are you? Are you female or male? When was the last time you ate? What was the last thing you ate? How strong is your digestive fire? There are countless factors that attribute and contribute to what your body needs to function optimally. Ultimately, you need to listen to how you feel and make decisions from there.

Here's an example. During my 3rd flare up foods that helped me recover during the first and second flare up only made it worse this time around. I had to stop using my previous recipe book, start from scratch, and go back to the drawing board again. With that in mind, I refuse to write a recipe section in this book.

Understanding the process of selecting food and

understanding what makes food good for us is very important to make educated decisions.

Take note of the way you eat your food and the way you prepare your food. Notice how this affects you. Take note of what is in your food. Do you know what additives are in your food and what they do to you?

You are what you eat
Diet matters... a lot

Everything you eat affects you, seriously. Every doctor I went to told me diet didn't matter. They told me there wasn't a specific diet that would help. Even the dietitian, who was a Crohn's Disease specialist, had no food advice for me. Through trial and error and keeping a food log, I found it's as simple as this, put junk food into your system and you will get poor health back. Put healthy organic foods into your system and you will become a healthy person.

Be mindful of what you are intolerant to eating. I found when flare up are active I could not tolerate most foods. As my digestion improved and my organs became stronger, I was able to consume a larger variety of foods. This allowed me to eat healthier foods that I could not eat before such as fruits and veggies.

Monitor your diet closely pay attention to the details of what you consume. Make changes to your diet gradually and intelligently. Focus on eating meals that do not cause pain or discomfort. Let some of your favorite meals that irritate your bowels go for now.

Once you are healthy again you may find that you

tolerate those foods better now. Then again, you may have found an alternative favorite meal that you like even better, that feels good more often.

Strive to eat more real food and less filler

I only consider things that grow from the earth and animals real food. Everything else is filler. As you eat more organic real food you enjoy, you will train your body to crave the real stuff more and the filler less. You will gain more nutrition from the same amount of food. You will feel better with less effort.

Choose foods that are as additive free as possible

Additives are what they add to your food. Various chemicals used to flavor the food, preserve it from bugs and bacteria, add coloring, synthetic vitamins, and sometimes known poisons. At the very least spend some time to learn about the various additives and what they do. Educate yourself learn about what you are putting in your body.

In my experience, the more chemical ingredients listed on the side of the package the unhealthier the food was for me. I found that the food items with the least amount of processing, chemicals, pesticides, sugars, coloring, etc, were easier to digest. Foods that had additives or preservatives always caused more problems than those that did not. Even packaged foods advertised as health foods like protein shakes, energy bars, vitamin waters may include additives, preservatives, and chemicals. My recommendation is to avoid anything unnatural or anything out of a box or package. This includes cereal, canned food, frozen dinners, soup in a cup, granola bars, chips, soda, and much more. Get the idea?

Eat real organic foods that you can tolerate. This is not a diet. It's a set of guidelines that you could adopt if you want optimal digestive health. With some practice this becomes a habit and a lifestyle.

Upgrade your diet gradually and intelligently

If you think to yourself, "I only like to eat bad foods," don't fret. Simply, pick one healthy food you enjoy and eat more of it more often. I find fruit to be fantastic because it is healthy and sweet. Make the change gradual and comfortable. Choose healthier foods you enjoy. Don't pick something just because you think you should eat it. Make sure you pick something you enjoy that is organic, real, and healthy.

In addition to eating more healthy food you enjoy,

also pick a food that you know is bad that you continue to eat anyway. Take note of how often you consume it. Then do your best to eat less of this food less often. Start with the reducing the intake of foods that are easier to remove from your diet. Substitute them with something similar and healthier

If you think to yourself, "yuck healthy food," you can experiment with new healthy foods that you haven't tried before. Branch out and try new foods. Try different melons, berries, leafy greens, or other assorted fruits and vegetables. Try different sources of food such as a farmer's market. There is so much variety out there you are bound to find something you enjoy.

Eat slowly and savor your food

Chewing your food and coating your food in saliva

are the first steps of the digestive process. To ensure maximum digestion make sure that the food is chewed finely before the food is passing through your intestines. Chew each mouthful 20-30 times or more, allow it to become soft and smooth in your mouth. As you do this think to yourself how great the food is and how the food is going to nourish your body. Be in the moment and savor every bite and be thankful for being able to eat your meal.

Only eat when you are in a calm relaxed state

Digestion is at its best when you are calm and relaxed. Eating while angry, fearful, or anxious hinders the digestive process. Take a moment to calm down, slow down, and relax before eating. Stop eating on the run. Don't eat and drive. Stop doing other activities while eating. Be mindful. Focus your mind on how much you enjoy the food and how well it will nourish your body. Being stressed out releases cortisol. Cortisol deactivates digestion.

Eat but only eat when you are hungry and Stop eating when you are full

Pay attention to how your body feels so you know when you have had enough food. Eat slower so you can feel yourself fill up. Avoid that bloated feeling or being so full it hinders you. Being this full hinders the digestive process. Leave empty space in your stomach to aid in the digestive process.

If you are often stuffed after eating make your food portions smaller. Get in the habit of serving your own portions and putting the exact amount of food you think you need on your plate. This will keep you from going back for seconds. Stop eating when you are satisfied, not stuffed full. When you get hungry again eat more food. At first, you may need to learn how much food you require but you will get better with practice and your internal awareness will grow.

Don't starve yourself either. If you are hungry please eat organic chemical free food. Make sure you are consuming food regularly. If you are having a flare up or not eating regularly, not eating when hungry may feel like a good option but you are robbing your body of nutrients and calories it needs to heal.

Eat for nutrition, not for flavor nor because you are under emotional stress. Don't eat to avoid problems. Breathe to process your stress.

For optimal digestion after eating, I found I like my belly to contain about one third food, one third water, and one third empty.

Most importantly, see yourself with kind eyes. Don't be hard on yourself. Allow some slack and make adjustments at a rate you can handle.

Don't eat before bedtime

When you eat matters. I recommend your last meal or snack to be 2-8 hours before bedtime depending on the severity of the flare up or condition your digestion may be in. Following this advice will help relieve a number of digestive ailments.

Before I adopted this rule, I would wake up throughout the night. About an hour or two before I wanted to wake up, I would get up to go to the bathroom. This first bathroom break of the day would typically take me 45 minutes. After cutting out late night snacking, I found it much easier to sleep through the night.

Many people suggest no eating after dark. This is a solid rule that can be followed. If you must snack at night because you are starving make sure it's something light that you can easily digest. I found bananas to be especially good for this. Learn how long it takes you to digest various foods so you can plan on your stomach being empty by bedtime.

Drink LOTS of mineral water

Drink water. Drink plenty of mineral water. I drink water 99% of the time. Your body is more than 50% water and you are perspiring all the time. Make sure you keep it replenished and with fresh clean mineral water.

For optimal functionality, the human body needs to drink mineral water regularly. Drink at least enough water to counter out the amount you are losing through excretion, perspiration, and the environment. This includes sweating due to physical activity levels, going to the bathroom, heat, and humidity of your environment. Then drink some more water to keep your body systems hydrated and lubricated.

Drink more water to help with bowel movements. Drinking water keeps everything flowing right. Anytime I feel backed up, I counter it with more water. Anytime it's a little liquidy, drink more water to counter the losses.

Larger people, this includes more height and more weight, need more water. Physically active people, need more water. If you are exercising, drink extra water to counter out the loss of fluids.

The feelings of dry eyes, chapped lips, or parched throat, are all indicators of dehydration and thirst. If you are thirsty your body is telling you it needs more water.

Anytime my urine is yellow, I gradually increase my water intake until it is nearly clear again.

During the day, I drink every time I think about water. You don't have to chug a cup of water every time you think of it, but at least take a sip. I think sipping water all day every day is one of the best things I did for my digestion.

I find drinking a large amount of water (16 oz+) in the morning really helps make the whole day go smoother. Throughout the day, I do my best to maintain regular consumption of water.

At night I drink a large amount of water (16 oz+) before bed. Drinking extra water before bed would provide me with enough water to make that first morning bowel movement go a lot smoother. If I didn't drink enough water, I would need to wake up an hour early to get that first bowel movement of the day going. It would be slow, painful, and loose, all at the same time. Drinking extra water at night (16+ oz) reduced about 5-15 minutes off my morning bathroom visit and allowed everything to flow more smoothly.

If you feel bloated or you feel water sloshing around in you, wait a while before drinking more water. Give your body time to absorb the fluid. Consuming a bit of salt helps water absorb.

Drink small amounts of water while eating because too much will dilute your system and slow down digestion making it less efficient and causing discomfort.

Consume some salt with your water

Salt is an essential electrolyte that directs the flow of fluid in our body. Eat some salt to help absorb the water. Some signs of needing more salt include excessive sweating, excessive peeing, waking up to pee in the middle of the night, diarrhea, and sweaty palms. Each time we pee, we flush all of our salt from our system.

Drinking tea has many benefits

To make tea soak herbs in boiling hot water for a few minutes. When the water changes colors it is infused with the herbs. Strain out the solid parts and enjoy.

Liquid's like tea do not need to be broken down in your body the same way as food. This allows your body to extract the nutrition with less effort. During flare ups, I enjoy drinking warm organic tea. My favorite teas made my guts feel better. Ginger, mint, or other herbs can assist in digestion. I find tea helps me most right after a meal, especially after a large meal or a cold meal. It helps soothe an achy belly and helps regulate my body temperature.

Tea makes a great healthy morning treat without filling your belly with heavy foods that may be harder to process. I enjoy tea before bed which would help me sleep better as well as quell my desire to snack.

Chapter 7:

This is a Lifestyle Change, Keep Doing the Work

Keep this new lifestyle going

Once you are able to restore your health, the next most important idea you can learn is how to avoid a relapse or backtracking. In my experience, there are a few key concepts that I suggest are worth paying attention to.

Tune in to yourself and develop self-awareness

Feel the physical sensations inside your body. Do you ache? Do you feel strong? What are the kinds of thoughts you are having? Are they positive? Are they negative? Are they confusing?

Observe the habits that you are performing. Are they beneficial? Do they represent the true inner you?

Pay attention to your thoughts and where they are coming from. Observe them. What are your thoughts telling you about your state of being?

Be truthful with yourself. See things objectively, as they really are.

Observe thoughts and processes before a relapse occurs

I noticed, when I would stop treating myself lovingly, I would become impatient with myself. I would ignore my positive thoughts, routines, and feelings that I have been developing. I was comfortable in returning to my old lifestyle.

As someone who is successfully recovering from digestion problems, I acknowledge negative recurring thoughts could throw me off track. Eating, thinking, or acting, unhealthy will eventually break down the body.

Note the feelings and sensations within before a relapse occurs

Quiet your mind. Feel deep inside. Note if you are

well.

Before a relapse, there are physical indicators and sensations that might indicate deteriorating health. Sensations may include:

- Increased intestinal pain or sensation.
- Increased spasms or cramps.
- Burning insides.
- Increased body temperature or fever.
- Trouble sleeping through the night.
- Increased urgency or frequency of bowel movements.

When inner feelings of pain rise to the surface, acknowledge and feel them. Do what feels right to soothe, heal, and rejuvenate.

Pace yourself and take breaks

After a day of unhealthy eating habits (feasting, eating cakes or desserts, stuffing myself, drinking soda or alcohol, eating foods that cause problems), I take the next day off of that and follow my good established routine as best as possible. No exceptions, all choices, that are hard on the body, require at least one full day of good choices to recover from.

If I don't feel better after a day of my good behavior, I take another day off and focus on good eating habits. Sometimes one day won't be enough to return to a positive feeling inside. If this is the case, keep repeating these good days until the body feels just right again.

Perform light exercise daily

Any kind of light activity is great to help prevent atrophy and keep the cells healthy and regenerating at an optimal level. Currently, I am doing yoga and isometrics for exercise. I am not doing anything very intense or high impact. If my guts are acting up at all, I enjoy a long slow walk 15 min to an hour or I practice gentle restorative yoga with props.

Drink more mineral water

Drinking water keeps everything flowing right. When I wake up in the morning and before I go to bed, I like to drink a big cup of water to cleanse my system of toxins. Throughout the day all day, I sip water.

Take notes and log your progress as a reminder

I encourage you to log everything that works. This will help remind you and keep you on track. Take note of every action that brings you closer to health. Keep track of all your actions, thoughts, habits, and foods that you respond well to. This way you can repeat them as often as possible. Leave reminders for yourself anywhere that helps. Keep track of the foods, actions, thoughts, habits that deter, hurt, or injure you so you can avoid them as often as possible.

This book started as just that. I started writing this book as advice for myself to help me during a relapse. When my first major relapse came in 2010, I returned to my own notes and read my advice. My own advice was so beneficial for myself I was able to get back on my feet faster than before.

Follow your dreams

Life is too short to live someone else's dreams. Being off track from your goals and dreams in life can cause huge ripples in your health. Be true to yourself to live life at its fullest and healthiest.

As momentum builds, the journey gets easier

With consistent progress, you will make it past the tipping point. Improvement will gradually become automatic and habitual. Results will gain momentum become more common in your reality. As you begin seeing improvements it gets easier to maintain where you are at because:

- You may have learned how to heal yourself to the point where you are at.

- You may have developed new habits and skills that will help you along the way.
- Your mindset may have changed to be more positive to the situation and more understanding to what is going on inside your body.

There is always room for improvement

I feel that there is no max to how healthy, strong, calm, balanced, and flexible you can become. These characteristics apply to both body and mind. The only limits are self-imposed. Don't get me wrong, there may be ups, downs, valleys, mountains, and plateaus. Know that things always change and the rate of progression changes too. I strive to improve and become stronger and healthier. Make it a lifelong commitment. It has been worth it for me.

It's OK to make mistakes

Don't beat yourself up for not being perfect. Human beings are perfect with all of their imperfections. No one is perfect all the time. Everyone makes mistakes in various areas of their lives. Use mistakes as learning experiences to grow from. Make corrections and keep going.

Have a support network of loving people

Surround yourself with good people who are looking out for you and encouraging you to better yourself.

Summary

- Decide that you can and will be healthy again.

- You get what you expect.

- Be positive.

- Always do your best and only your best.

- Reduce negative influences in your life.

- Eat healthy organic clean food.

- Perform some daily physical activity.

- Breathe long and deep often.

- Drink plenty of water.

- Eat a well-balanced nutritious diet.

- Listen to your body and feel the sensations within.

- Take time to recuperate between unhealthy meals and activities.

- Get plenty of sleep to recover.

- Be objective. See things as they really are.

Not as you wish them to be.

- Everything changes.
- Never give up.